Clean Eating

The Comprehensive Manual For Establishing A Flourishing Food Delivery Enterprise Focused On Clean Eating

(The Comprehensive Manual On Maintaining A Clean Diet With Additional Culinary Recommendations And Dietary Outline)

Marty Herring

TABLE OF CONTENT

What Is The Definition Of Dietary Fiber? Why Is It Important?

Dietary fiber originates from plant-based sources, such as whole grains, fruits, and vegetables. It constitutes the portion of plant-derived nourishment that is not readily digested or absorbed by the human body. You might be curious regarding the indigestibility of fiber and its minimal contribution to the overall calorie intake. Consequently, what role does it perform within the human body? The reality is that a diet abundant in fiber can yield remarkable outcomes - the advantages encompass everything from promoting regular bowel movements, promoting a feeling of fullness, reducing the likelihood of excessive food consumption, managing body weight, to reducing cholesterol levels and moderating the body's blood glucose response following a meal. In fact, an abundance of scientific evidence has prompted numerous prestigious health organizations worldwide to endorse health claims regarding the benefits of fiber.

There exist two variants of fiber, one being soluble and the other insoluble, and both hold considerable significance. Both variants can be found in a particular food item, however, certain foods may serve as a more optimal source for either component. Soluble fiber has the ability to create a gel-like substance within the body, thereby causing a possible delay in gastric emptying. It is commonly recognized for its capacity to reduce cholesterol levels and facilitate the growth of beneficial bacteria. Insoluble fiber has the capacity to absorb water and increase volume, thereby facilitating the expeditious movement of waste through the body, ultimately contributing to the prevention of constipation.

Soluble fiber can be found in a variety of food sources, including barley, oats, nuts, legumes such as rajma and channa, peas, apples, pears, and flax seeds. Insoluble fiber can be found in various whole grain cereals such as wheat bran and whole wheat flour, as well as in foods like brown rice, nuts, seeds, dates, and vegetables.

The majority of individuals aspire to lead prolonged and robust lives. Due to this circumstance, numerous individuals are inclined to modify their dietary habits and daily routines in order to increase the likelihood of achieving this outcome. One possible modification that could prove beneficial is the incorporation of a greater amount of dietary fiber into one's nutritional intake. This area holds significant importance, as it is commonly observed that numerous individuals have deficiencies in their dietary habits, which can be readily rectified through the adoption of a sensible eating regime.

Dietary fiber possesses several noteworthy advantages. Initially, it can aid in weight reduction as it induces a sensation of satiety while consuming fibrous substances, consequently resulting in reduced food intake. It can additionally assist in reducing cholesterol levels and potentially act as a preventive measure against certain types of cancer, such as colon cancer.

There are two primary categories of dietary fiber found in food, each of which imparts distinct benefits. The two categories encompass soluble fiber and insoluble fiber. Flora comprises both varieties of fiber, albeit in varying proportions contingent upon the botanical species.

If one desires to consume a diet abundant in soluble fiber, it is necessary to include fruits, vegetables, lentils, beans, and akin items in their meals. If you are inclined to consume insoluble fiber, it would be advisable to incorporate food options like brown rice and wholemeal bread into your diet. In addition, fruits and vegetables also comprise a generous amount of both insoluble and soluble dietary fiber.

It is crucial to ensure adequate fluid intake, comprising water, tea, coffee, or low-calorie squash, while consuming fibrous foods to facilitate their optimal functionality. Food fiber has the capacity to absorb water in a manner similar to that of a sponge. It increases in size as it absorbs the water within the stomach, thereby facilitating the sensation of satiety.

Many food items that possess a significant amount of dietary fiber tend to have a reduced fat content. The exceptions pertain to seeds and nuts. According to current guidelines, it is recommended that the average adult intake approximately eighteen grams of fiber daily. However, it should be noted that this recommendation is currently being reviewed and there is a possibility that it may be raised to a maximum of thirty grams per day. In the United Kingdom, the average individual consumes a mere twelve grams daily, a quantity that is deemed insufficient.

Dietary fiber aids in the reduction of blood cholesterol levels. It additionally aids in maintaining stable blood glucose and insulin levels, thereby constituting a significant factor in mitigating the risk associated with cardiovascular disease and type 2 diabetes.

Individuals afflicted with diverticulitis, hemorrhoids, and constipation can also experience alleviation of their symptoms and a reduction in complications by adopting a dietary regimen that is abundant in dietary fiber. Fiber significantly aids in the regulation of your digestive system, preventing the occurrence of constipation.

Dietary fiber is exclusively present in plant-based foods. Canned and frozen produce retains an equivalent amount of dietary fiber compared to fresh produce. Nonetheless, the elimination of seeds or the peeling of the produce will result in a diminishment of the dietary fiber content present in the food.

Considering that these foods serve as the foundation of a nourishing diet and encompass various elements with exceptional nutritional value, such as vitamins, minerals, and phytochemicals, it would be advantageous to consume a greater quantity of them, irrespective of the supplementary advantages derived from their fiber content.

An evident approach to incorporating fiber into your daily dietary intake is by consuming it during the morning alongside your breakfast. If one commences the morning meal with a serving of nutritious cereal choices such as whole wheat biscuits, corn flakes, or porridge, there is a significant improvement in the overall fiber consumption.

However, numerous breakfast cereals that are currently popular exhibit cunning in their presentation. They possess a significant abundance of sugars while frequently exhibiting considerably lower levels of dietary fiber than one might envision. Examine the packaging of your preferred 'sweet cereal' and juxtapose it with that of a more simplistic variation. The numbers will leave you astounded. If you or your child desires a sweet or fruit-flavored breakfast cereal, it is advisable to opt for the unsweetened variant and enhance its flavor by adding freshly cut fruit. It exhibits exquisite flavor, while simultaneously providing a notable dose of dietary fiber, thus offering a nourishing and healthful morning meal.

Whilst there exist supplements that can be utilized to augment your consumption of dietary fiber, it is advisable to prioritize obtaining fiber from whole food sources. Firstly, one does not obtain the additional benefits associated with consuming the food, and furthermore, these benefits may not prove as advantageous for various other reasons.

These supplements may potentially interact with certain medications you may be currently prescribed, whereas food consumption would not pose a similar concern. Furthermore, various varieties of fiber can be found in different foods. However, the specific benefits provided by each type remain unclear, thus it is possible that consuming a supplement with the incorrect type of fiber could result in missing out on the desired benefits.

One additional justification for consuming dietary fiber through the consumption of vegetables and fruits as opposed to relying on a dietary supplement is that they contribute to the visual appeal of any culinary preparation, thereby promoting a wholesome and pleasurable dining experience.

Lastly, it is important to bear in mind the recommendations regarding the consumption of five servings of fruits or vegetables per day. Now that you comprehend the rationale behind this advice, you can appreciate its validity. Dietary fiber promotes overall well-being, diminishes cholesterol levels, and contributes to maintaining cardiovascular health. It can aid in weight reduction and diminish the likelihood of developing diabetes. Dietary fiber is undeniably a miraculous component in our food, one that should be further explored and acknowledged for its invaluable significance.

Quick Tip 3

Incorporating a generous quantity of cruciferous vegetables, including members such as broccoli, kale, and tomatoes, into the diet. Incorporating dietary modifications can be advantageous in counteracting the proliferation of cancer.

Plays an essential role in upholding mental well-being

In addition to the extensive advantages that maintaining a healthy diet confers upon one's physical well-being, it has been discovered to be highly beneficial for supporting mental well-being as well.

Certain essential nutrients found in a wholesome diet, such as vitamin B-6 commonly present in foods like banana and lean poultry, contribute to the synthesis of dopamine. This neurotransmitter plays a pivotal role in promoting feelings of well-being and enhancing mood. Furthermore, it has been discovered that vital nutrients such as Omega-3 fatty acids also play a significant role in maintaining positive mental well-being. Therefore, a deficiency of these nutrients in the body could potentially lead to feelings of sadness and depression.

Quick Tip 4

• Limiting your consumption of caffeine can potentially enhance your mental well-being, as excessive intake has been linked to increased anxiety levels.

• Additionally, it is imperative that you refrain from missing meals as doing so can potentially result in heightened levels of stress, headaches, or abdominal discomfort.

A Healthy Skin

The act of consuming wholesome food in order to preserve a luminous complexion and appear healthy has been an enduring tradition that can even be traced back to biblical times, specifically when the Jewish people were in exile in Babylon. Daniel and his companions had chosen to adhere to a wholesome dietary regimen comprising of fruits, legumes, vegetables, and water, instead of partaking from the provisions provided at the King's table. Following the conclusion of the trial, it was determined that Daniel and his companions possessed a superior state of well-being and a more refined appearance compared to their counterparts who had opted for sustenance from the royal table.

The enduring wisdom of that pivotal lesson remains highly relevant in our present era. It is worth emphasizing that adhering to a regimen characterized by the avoidance of processed foods, empty calories, refined sugar, and excessive alcohol consumption will undoubtedly yield a resplendent, luminous complexion. The rationale behind this is that these detrimental factors have a tendency to deprive the skin of numerous essential nutrients necessary to maintain its resilience and elasticity. Certainly, one can enhance the appearance of their skin by replenishing it with vital nutrients obtained through the consumption of whole foods abundant in skin-boosting compounds such as beneficial fats and potent antioxidants.

You will experience an astonishing depth of flavor in your culinary creations." "Your food is imbued with an extraordinary level of taste and flavor." "The flavors in your dishes are truly remarkable, surpassing expectations.

Consuming a nutritious diet entails the incorporation of a well-balanced assemblage of natural foods comprising wholesome proteins, carbohydrates, spices, and fats. Upon embarking on the adoption of this particular lifestyle, you shall undoubtedly be astounded by the unparalleled sensory experience that accompanies the consumption of unprocessed edibles, for you shall truly savor the authentic essence of natural sustenance.

The vast majority of food items found within the conventional American diet contain a plethora of chemical additives such as stabilizers, preservatives, and sweeteners, which often serve to mask the inherent flavors of these culinary offerings. The outcome of these substances is such that they have a tendency to leave a lingering taste that could become perceptible as your palate adjusts to consuming organic, unadulterated food.

In addition to the enhanced energy levels, decrease in gastrointestinal discomfort, and overall improved sense of well-being that accompany this lifestyle, you will find that your culinary experiences are exponentially enhanced and surpassed by what you once envisioned. Importantly, as you progressively limit your consumption of unhealthy foods, the allure of craving them will significantly diminish, leading you to experience the true flavors of wholesome foods and instilling a sense of gratitude for such nourishment.

Maintaining a Nutritious Diet Does Not Have to Be Costly

When contrasting the significant financial impact of dining out at restaurants, ordering takeout, and indulging in unhealthy snacks, it becomes evident that preparing nutritious and delicious meals at home not only proves cost-effective, but also emerges as a superior choice. Furthermore, through careful strategic planning, it is possible to acquire necessary food provisions at affordable prices from nearby farmers' markets, natural foods stores, or cooperatives, thus enabling one to adhere to a clean eating regimen without incurring significant costs.

Aids in the Reduction of Excessive Body Weight" "Facilitates the Reduction of Excess Weight" "Assists in Achieving a

Decrease in Body Weight" "Supports the Attainment of a Healthy Body Weight

By integrating appropriate exercise regimens, dietary supplements, and adhering to a wholesome eating regimen, one is bound to achieve the desired physique and form within a short span of time, accompanied by numerous advantageous outcomes.

Clean Eating Benefits

You may contemplate the recent surge of interest in adopting a clean eating lifestyle, and what precisely constitutes this notion.

In essence, it denotes consuming foods in their most unadulterated form, or as close to their natural state as feasible. Given that individuals are now aware of the negative effects that excessive consumption of additives and chemicals can have on their bodies over an extended period, they are actively seeking methods to eliminate these substances from their diets and purify their bodies. By doing so, they aim to achieve a state of greater equilibrium and stability in their overall health. This is why the concept of adhering to a clean eating regimen has gained widespread popularity in the current period. Consuming a wholesome diet entails the consumption of nourishing food. The smaller the number of additives present in food, the more closely it adheres to its natural state and exhibits superior quality. The higher the number of ingredients in food, the greater the extent of food processing and the increased presence of additives and chemicals. Consuming a wholesome diet entails the consumption of unprocessed and nourishing foods such as fruits, vegetables, lean proteins, and complex carbohydrates. It also entails refraining from consuming unhealthy food. Processed food refers to comestibles comprising artificial sweeteners, unhealthy fats (hydrogenated, trans-fat), preservatives, and refined flour. Junk food is abundant in empty calories and lacks any significant nutritional value.

The primary focus of the clean eating program does not solely revolve around weight loss, but rather emphasizes maximizing overall health and wellness. This is the rationale behind why adopting a clean eating regimen transcends mere fad status and embodies a long-term lifestyle choice. The subject matter pertains to examining sustenance as a source of energy for the human body, rather than simply considering food as a means to satisfy physiological needs. Eating clean is not simply a dietary regimen aimed at overcoming difficulties, but rather a method of enhancing one's well-being. The goal is to create a foundation from which one can develop a strong character and physique. In contrast to a diet, there is no concern about relapsing as it entails a permanent change in your overall dietary habits.

Consuming a reduced quantity of food aids in the pursuit of physical fitness as it has the effect of decreasing metabolic rate rather than enhancing it. Consuming a reduced amount of carbohydrates and depriving the body of necessary nutrients will lead to instability in glucose levels, thereby increasing cravings for unhealthy food choices. An additional adverse effect of refraining from food is muscle loss due to the incapacity of stored fat to be converted into glucose, leading the body to resort to breaking down muscle tissue to provide energy through glucose.

Presently, health professionals adhere to this regimen of consuming wholesome food through three distinct approaches. The technique you select should be based on your individual body type and lifestyle. As an illustration, there are individuals who merely require consuming the same three customary meals daily, yet they aim to eliminate processed foods from their diet. Other individuals may need to adhere to a regimen that enhances their metabolism and stabilizes their blood glucose levels, thus following option two, which currently holds the highest degree of popularity. Individuals with concerns about developing diabetes due to family history typically opt for the third approach.

"The recommended guidelines for The Eating Clean Projects include:

• Eliminate the consumption of processed sugar.

• Engage in the act of perusing the names of food items and consuming sustenance that possess a lesser number of ingredients (endeavor to abstain from consuming nourishment products that consist of more than 3-6 ingredients).

• Prepare and consume nutritious meals to avoid making impulsive unhealthy choices.

• Ensure proper hydration by consuming a daily intake of eight glasses of water.

• Eliminate the provision of mixed refreshments (or alternatively, completely restrict it).

• Dependably have breakfast.

Incorporate an ample variety of fruits and vegetables into your dietary regime.

• Substitute white sugars with cocoa or whole grains such as chestnut rice, for example. Both whole wheat pasta and whole wheat bread are viable options.

• Rest, Physical Activity, Stress Management: Strive to maintain a consistent sleep schedule of 7 to 8 hours. Various sectors such as rest, physical exercise, hydration, essential nutrients, and stress management should all collaborate in order to enhance internal equilibrium.

• The inclusion of protein in your diet is crucial as it prompts the release of the hormone glucagon (which elevates glucose levels), thereby counterbalancing the hormone insulin (known for lowering glucose levels). As a result, a balanced interplay between these two hormones occurs, leading to stable blood sugar levels. Protein serves as the foremost factor facilitating the development, restoration, and maintenance of bodily tissue. Complete protein can be sourced from dietary options such as poultry (chicken, turkey), fish, beef, and other meats.

• Consume foods rich in dietary fiber: Incorporating dietary fiber into your diet is crucial as it cannot be digested, thus effectively slowing down the rate of digestion and aiding in optimal blood glucose regulation. The aim is to consume a daily intake of 25-35 grams of fiber.

• Consume Optimal Unsaturated Fats rather than Detrimental Saturated Fats: Fat itself is not the enemy; however, excessive consumption of saturated fats can lead to health issues. The benefits of consuming unsaturated fat include retarding absorption, promoting the release of stored fats, facilitating the utilization of fat-soluble vitamins, and providing essential fatty acids.

"Food items to Avoid or Minimize to the Greatest Extent Possible:

• Sugar

• Confections (pastries, sweet treats, baked goods)

• Cheddar

• Chilled yogurt

• Mayonnaise

• Crisps

• Pop

• Bread

• Meals that come already prepared, such as pre-stuffed dinners or box-based items like pop tarts, oats, frozen entrees, cookies, and pasta, are not allowed.

• Avoid consuming saturated fats that elevate your cholesterol levels and enhance the risk of coronary artery disease (fatty meat, whole milk, bacon, butter, cheese, ice cream)

•   Combine small quantities of unsaturated fats such as avocados, olives, and canola oil.

•   Partially hydrogenated oils (an ingredient added to foods in order to extend their shelf life)

• Assess the sodium content in food. • Verify the sodium levels in food. • Examine the sodium concentration in food. • Evaluate the sodium quantity in food. • Scrutinize the sodium levels in food. The presence of sodium in food, specifically in each gram (1000mg) of sodium, leads to the retention of water molecules in the body, resulting in bloating and swelling, and adversely affecting the functioning of the digestive system. The goal is to limit your sodium intake to a range of 1,500 to 2,000.

Great Nourishments:

• Chicken

• Eggs

• Dairy

• Soy-based products

- Animal protein, recreational activity

- Assorted nuts and seeds

- Fish

- Turkey Breast

- Greek style yogurt

Unsaturated fats are allowed.

- Coconut, seed-derived oils such as olive oil and flaxseed oil, and natural spreads

THREE Approaches TO ADOPT FOR MAINTAINING A HEALTHY DIET

Plan 1

Abstain from consuming processed foods of various kinds, and instead adhere to the customary three meals per day (Breakfast, Lunch, and Dinner).

Strategy 2

Consensus among wellness experts suggests that in order to achieve weight loss, it is advisable to increase one's food intake. This program relies on a dietary plan consisting of organic foods ingested through multiple meals throughout the day. Following this approach to dietary consumption helps regulate your blood sugar levels and maintain overall bodily equilibrium. In addition to purging your system of incorporated chemicals and additives, adhering to a clean diet also entails the benefit of weight reduction. Nourishment that undergoes increased handling is subject to expedited processing and may result in elevated glucose levels. Nourishment that is closer to its natural state requires less time for preparation, and slower digestion leads to improved glucose stability. Glucose reliability is associated with an elevated metabolic rate, leading to increased fat burning and overall bodily equilibrium. The rationale behind the importance of maintaining equilibrium in the body's glucose levels is due to the fact that when glucose levels are low, the body initiates intense cravings for glucose, leading to cravings for carbohydrates, as glucose is derived from sugars. Consuming only three meals a day can lead to a disrupted digestive system and elevated blood glucose levels, subsequently increasing the likelihood of consuming unhealthy meals. The most effective strategy to monitor your physiological cravings for nourishment is to maintain stable glucose levels throughout the day. "When you adhere to this methodology, you should:

• Adhere to the program's formula, which relies on correctly measuring the calorie intake per meal and ensuring appropriate nutrient proportions (40% protein, 25% fats, 35% carbohydrates), to regulate glucose levels based on overall body composition and lean body mass (LBM). The extent of calories expended is contingent upon whether one aims to maintain, reduce, or increase their weight. As an example, in the case where a woman desires to achieve weight loss, it is recommended that she consumes approximately 250 calories per meal, while a man should consume 400 calories per meal, spaced out every 3 to 4 hours. If the aim is to achieve weight gain and enhance muscle definition, it is recommended that women consume approximately 300 calories and men consume 500 calories every 3 to 4 hours until their desired weight is achieved. Maintaining weight is optimally achieved between these two extremes.

• Consume a well-balanced meal every 3 to 4 hours (consisting of five to six smaller portioned meals per day).

Strategy 3

The third method is endorsed by Jillian Michaels, an esteemed authority in wellness and the renowned figure from "The Biggest Loser" television show.

This methodology entails adopting a comparable approach to "clean eating," while restricting one's meals to only four per day. In this approach, it is suggested to adhere to a regular eating schedule rather than consuming meals at intervals of 2-3 hours. The underlying premise of this methodology posits that maintaining a consistent eating pattern, as opposed to frequent meals every 2-3 hours, can help individuals avoid the persistent spiking of insulin levels and thereby mitigate the potential risk of developing diabetes.

Pan-Seared Chicken With A Curry-Infused Apricot Glaze, Served With Broccoli And Almonds.

Ingredients:

- ¼ cup of Dry White Wine

- ¾ Cup of Chicken Broth - Low Sodium

- 2 Tbsp. of Raw Honey

- Zest from ½ Orange

- 2 Tbsp of Unsalted, Organic Butter - Diced

- ¼ Cup of unsalted, Slivered Almonds

- 4 - 5 ounce Chicken Breasts - Boneless and Skinless

- ⅛ tsp. of Sea Salt

- ⅛ tsp. of Pepper

- 3 Tbsp. of Olive Oil - Divided

- 2 Bunches of Broccoli - Trimmed

- 4 Green Fresh onions - Chopped, Divided

- 2 Tbsp. of Ginger - Minced

- 2 Tbsp. of Garlic - Minced - divided

- 2 tsp. Of Curry Powder

- ½ tsp. of Red Pepper Flakes

- 4 Cups of Sliced Apricots - 8 Apricots

Instructions:

• Please ensure that your oven is preheated to a temperature of 400 degrees Fahrenheit.

Enhance the flavor of your chicken by sprinkling ⅛ teaspoon of seasoning. of salt and pepper. In a large pan on high heat, heat up 2 tbsp. of oil. Incorporate the chicken and proceed to sear it until it attains a browned texture on both sides. It is estimated that the duration of this task will be approximately four minutes. Invert it and proceed to relocate it to a baking dish for subsequent cooking in the oven. Ensure the roast is thoroughly cooked by exposing it to heat until done. It is estimated that it will require approximately 10 minutes. Relocate it onto a dish and cover it with a foil tent.

• Simmer the broccoli in a pot of boiling water until it reaches a tender consistency. The estimated duration of this task is approximately 3 to 4 minutes. Remove the liquid and subsequently transfer it to the ice water for the purpose of cooling. Empty it once more and set it aside.

Incorporate the whites of the green fresh onions and ginger into the same pan with the chicken drippings over medium heat, adding 1 tablespoon. Comprised of garlic, curry powder, and a sprinkle of pepper flakes. Continue cooking it until the fresh onions have reached a tender consistency. The estimated duration is approximately one minute.

• Incorporate the apricots into the mixture; raise the heat to medium-high. Place the lid on the pan and proceed to sauté it for a duration of 3 minutes. Incorporate the wince into the process and dislodge the browned residue from the pan employing a wooden spoon. After the wine has dissipated, carefully incorporate the broth into the mixture. Add in the honey and the orange zest. Continue cooking the dish until the sauce reaches the desired state of thickness. The task is projected to require a time frame of approximately five to six minutes.

• Incorporate the butter until it forms an emulsion. Incorporate the fresh onion greens into the mixture, seasoning it with a pinch of salt and a pinch of pepper. Ensure its warmth by placing a cover over it.

• In a generously sized skillet over medium heat, incorporate 1 tablespoon. of oil. Add in 1 tbsp. Sauté until fragrant, for approximately 30 seconds. Incorporate the broccoli and heat it until warmed through. The estimated duration for completion is three minutes. Stir in the almonds and additional salt and pepper. Presently apply the sauce atop the chicken and serve the broccoli alongside.

Sourcing Your Ingredients

An imperative inquiry that arises when the concept of clean eating is broached pertains to the origin of one's ingredients. I would be pleased to demonstrate to you the methods and locations through which you can obtain the finest quality ingredients for your culinary endeavors.

One notable establishment worth mentioning is the longstanding farmer's market. Due to the emergence of prominent chain supermarkets, the prevalence of farmer's markets has significantly diminished. Fortunately for you, this also signifies that they adopt a competitive pricing strategy and endeavor to provide their customers with the utmost quality in their products. It is probable that the typical vendor at a farmer's market possesses awareness of the health-conscious nature of their customer base, and thus aims to offer clean and unprocessed ingredients.

Peruse the pages of your community newspaper, particularly during the onset of Spring and the culmination of Summer, to gather information regarding nearby markets and events. Acquire knowledge regarding the harvest schedules in your vicinity in order to determine the appropriate periods for monitoring the availability of your preferred ingredients. You can derive a sense of satisfaction from the fact that you have contributed to the sustenance of a local enterprise.

Engaging in meaningful conversations with the individuals responsible for cultivating the food that is being sold can significantly contribute to easing any concerns regarding the trajectory of our food, right from its origin in the fields to its presence on our dining tables. Kindly inquire about any matters that may be of concern to you, whether it pertains to the origin of the seeds or the utilization of pesticides. You may acquire considerable knowledge about the craft too!

In reference to that, one can establish the precise origins of their food by engaging in the act of cultivating it personally. For the majority of individuals, engaging in extensive agricultural practices is impractical, yet individuals ranging from residents of apartments and trailers to land-owning ranchers possess the opportunity to cultivate plant life to some extent. Even hanging in a window, it is feasible to cultivate tomato plants in an inverted manner.

By making a modest investment, you have the opportunity to cultivate select crops and diligently care for them, thus ensuring a reliable supply of delectable sustenance. Tomatoes, as previously mentioned, enjoy widespread popularity. A substantial number of individuals residing in the United States' Southern region cultivate their own squash and peppers.

By engaging in the practice of composting your food waste, you will acquire a highly beneficial soil amendment that can greatly enhance the growth and yield of various crops. Ensure that you acquaint yourself with the prerequisites for each plant, encompassing their optimal growth climate, soil requirements, cultivation practices, and pest management. Cultivating your own produce can be highly fulfilling and has the potential to substantially decrease your expenses.

Basic Nutrition Guide

To adhere to a lifestyle of consuming nutritious foods, it is necessary to acquire substantial knowledge pertaining to various food items and their comprehensive impact on one's physical well-being. Though it may appear to be a daunting task initially, once you acquaint yourself with its fundamental principles, you will come to recognize that adopting a clean eating regimen becomes effortlessly inherent.

Reading Labels

Given that it is difficult to completely abstain from consuming processed foods, it is of utmost importance that you acquaint yourself with the fundamental tenets of comprehending nutritional information provided on product labels. Nonetheless, considering the wide array of culinary options available, I will merely address a limited selection of guidelines to initiate you.

If one lacks experience in culinary pursuits, they may tend to evaluate the cleanliness of their meals based on the quantity of ingredients used. In the initial chapter, it has been noted that food containing over six ingredients does not meet the criteria of being deemed clean. Nevertheless, there exist cases that deviate from this established principle. For instance, in the event that a food product consists of a total of 15 ingredients, yet all of them adhere to organic or fresh standards, it remains eligible for classification as a nutritious and uncontaminated food item.

Now, in the event that you are in search of pre-packaged edibles such as sauces and similar items, it would be advisable to carefully peruse the product's label to ascertain the specific ingredients employed in its production. Packaged foods that meet the criteria of being clean are those containing ingredients that can be purchased individually.

Consider pre-packaged broths as an illustrative instance. Upon examining the label and observing the presence of the ingredients "vegetable broth, salt, pepper," it can be deduced that the product qualifies as a sanitary pre-packaged component, given that both salt and pepper can be separately purchased and utilized alongside homemade vegetable broth. In the event that the packaging displays the ingredients as "vegetable broth, salt, pepper, monosodium glutamate," it is advisable to explore alternative options.

Kindly note, refrain from purchasing products that include any components with scientific-sounding names. It could prove somewhat challenging to locate wholesome food options, however, if your intention is to prepare nutritious meals, it would be most advisable to procure fresh ingredients and engage in home cooking. Individuals who adhere to a clean eating lifestyle are typically individuals who derive great pleasure from culinary activities. Therefore, if one's intention is to adhere to a healthy diet, it is imperative to acquire the skills needed to prepare nutritious meals.

On Eating More

Clean eating promotes the consumption of meals or snacks at a frequency of 5 to 6 times per day. This does not imply that it is necessary to consume a greater amount of food on a daily basis. Instead, it entails dividing your regular daily food intake into 5 to 6 smaller portions. It is advisable to maintain a daily caloric intake within acceptable parameters, ensuring a gap of two to three hours after a meal before consuming additional food. As an illustration, it is possible to establish a designated time slot for consuming a snack, preferably between 2 and 3 hours subsequent to each main meal. By doing so, you will maintain your health and vitality throughout the course of the day.

If you have concerns regarding portion sizes, you may begin by preparing a quantity of food that aligns with your typical daily intake, and subsequently divide it into five or six individual portions. An alternative approach would be to utilize your hands as a reliable means for gauging the proportions of your meal. A recommended portion size corresponds to the dimensions of one's hand's palm.

When determining portions for fruits and grains, simply enclose your hand into a cup-like shape, which constitutes an adequate single serving. When selecting portions of meat, it is advisable to observe the size of your hand placed palm-down, as this represents a single serving size.

Lastly, with regards to vegetables, a single serving is equivalent to the volume that can be contained within two cupped hands. By employing this approach, one will be spared from speculative estimations of serving proportions. It is equally crucial to engage in meal planning to prevent excessive calorie intake while following this diet.

Fiber, Cholesterol, and Sodium

Given that clean eating entails the consumption of copious amounts of food and vegetables, it is advisable to closely monitor your daily fiber intake. The consumption of a sizable amount of dietary fibers leads to dehydration and the depletion of crucial minerals in the body. The prescribed daily fiber intake is 14g for every 1000 calories of food ingested. For the ordinary individual adhering to a typical dietary regimen, the recommended daily intake of fiber falls within the range of 25 grams to 35 grams.

Fiber can be obtained from a variety of sources, such as fresh and dried fruits, uncooked vegetables, cereals and breads made from whole grains, legumes, and the edible peels of fruits and vegetables.

The maximum permissible daily intake for cholesterol is 300mg, as per the recommended guidelines. Given that clean eating emphasizes the consumption of fresh ingredients, it facilitates the effective management of cholesterol intake. With regards to sodium, the recommended daily intake limit is 2300mg per day. Nevertheless, if you possess a medical condition, it is advisable to adhere to the guidance provided by your physician.

Proteins

The amount of protein that an individual needs to consume varies based on their weight, resulting in a different recommended daily allowance for each person. To ascertain the optimal daily protein intake, it is advisable to calculate the product of your weight in kilograms and 0.8. It is vital to note that this particular equation is solely applicable to adult individuals maintaining a healthy weight. The calculation methods employed for individuals in the child and adolescent age groups differ.

If you are observing excessive weight, it is advisable to consider utilizing an intermediary weight value that lies between your present weight and the weight you aim to achieve. For instance, in the event that your current body weight is 90kg and your desired weight is 70kg, it is advisable to substitute 80kg in the equation in order to avoid subjecting your body to sudden deprivation of protein.

Should you be a bodybuilder, athlete, or in possession of a medical condition necessitating heightened protein intake, it is permissible to do so. As previously mentioned, this formula adheres to the established guidelines for individuals who are of typical health and wellbeing. Create a dietary plan focused on clean eating that aligns with the specific requirements of your body and lifestyle. Please be mindful of maintaining a proper balance of dietary ratios, as consuming excessive amounts of protein can lead to adverse effects, including but not limited to osteoporosis, cardiovascular diseases, cancer, obesity, and kidney stones.

Simplifying The Process Of Establishing Long And Short-Term Goals

In the pursuit of any alternative undertaking, it is crucial to establish objectives. Lacking objectives, one's path becomes ambiguous and unfocused. In regard to the concept of maintaining a healthy diet, it is imperative that individuals establish both immediate and long-term objectives, all of which should not only be clearly defined and quantifiable, but also attainable.

The primary issue leading to the failure of individuals in adhering to diets or making lifestyle changes can be attributed to their unrealistic expectations for rapid outcomes without being willing to invest the necessary amount of effort. Despite the presence of a convenient clean eating diet plan, failure to engage in thorough grocery shopping or home food preparation will not contribute to achieving improved health and well-being.

As mentioned earlier, there is no immediate need to initiate substantial modifications. You have the possibility to incorporate more nutritious meals into your current dietary regimen and build upon this foundation. Regarding your immediate objectives, it may involve the moderation of your fast food consumption, transitioning from a daily frequency to occurring only a few times per week. Progressively decrease this quantity as you proceed.

Alternatively, you could consider substituting your current practice of consuming one cookie per meal with the option of having a single cookie as a midday snack. There are minor adjustments that one can initiate in order to facilitate the long-term process of improving dietary choices for the body. As you advance with the integration, you can then direct your attention towards enduring objectives such as incorporating a consistent daily exercise routine or achieving a specific weight reduction within a predetermined timeframe.

Once more, it is crucial to clearly articulate your specific goals and intentions in relation to improving your dietary habits. Establish achievable objectives and encourage self-motivation to initiate action. The notion of "no pain, no gain" is not conducive to the mindset that you should adopt. Please take into consideration that a sufficient level of dedication is required in order to achieve favorable outcomes.

Opting For Nutritious Food Options

Opting for nutritional and hygienic food choices on a daily basis is of utmost significance. In order to accomplish this, it is imperative that you possess a fundamental comprehension of discerning what constitutes quality cuisine.

Beneficial Carbohydrates versus Detrimental Carbohydrates

Carbohydrates play a vital role as they serve as exceptional reservoirs of energy. However, it is important to note that excessively consuming carbohydrates on a regular basis should be avoided, as it can result in significant weight gain.

Similar to other constituents of food, there exist carbohydrates that are beneficial and carbohydrates that are detrimental. Gaining clarity on the distinction between these factors will enable you to make more informed dietary decisions while progressing towards a regimen focused on wholesome consumption. In essence, the unfavorable carbohydrates consist of the simple carbohydrates - sources of carbohydrates that are readily assimilated by your body immediately upon consumption. High-quality carbohydrates are complex in nature, requiring a more extended period for the body to metabolize. As a result, they provide a sustained and continuous supply of energy throughout the course of the day.

Substandard carbohydrates are detrimental due to their limited potential for metabolic breakdown. Alternatively, they undergo immediate processing and subsequent storage as adipose tissue. They fail to provide sustained satiation, leading to increased consumption in order to meet one's energy needs. These are the carbohydrates that are commonly present in white bread, pasta, and processed food.

Regarding complex carbohydrates, these can be obtained from sources such as whole grains and legumes. They provide satiety, resulting in an extended sensation of fullness. Furthermore, these also provide you with exceptional sources of dietary fiber. They do possess a certain level of sugar content, albeit not significantly high. An advantageous aspect lies in the fact that your body expends effort to appropriately digest and metabolize them. In addition, they also contribute to an increase in your metabolic rate, thereby facilitating gradual weight loss over time.

Differentiating between Beneficial and Detrimental Fats

The majority of individuals lack comprehension regarding the essence of adipose tissue, primarily due to its association with malignancies such as cholesterol, cardiovascular ailments, stroke, obesity, and even neoplastic conditions. However, it must be acknowledged that there exist specific types of fats that contribute to the proper functionality of the human body.

With regards to any dietary regimen, it is crucial to ensure a sufficient intake of beneficial fats into the body. There are certain foods that should be avoided or consumed in moderation, while there are also specific varieties that are necessary for attaining optimal health.

In essence, trans and saturated fats represent the two primary categories of unhealthy fats. The foremost organ affected by these substances is the heart, progressively becoming obstructed as their consumption escalates.

Saturated fats are animal-based. In addition to dairy products, high-fat cuts of meat also offer a source of these nutrients. In contrast, trans fats can be described as trans fatty acids derived from vegetable oils that have undergone partial hydrogenation. Trans fats are commonly found in processed food products like margarine, baked goods, and fast food items.

Nevertheless, it is important to bear in mind the existence of favorable fats. These contribute to improved cardiovascular health. Illustrations include polyunsaturated fat and monounsaturated fat. These types of fats, in contrast to their unhealthy counterparts, maintain a liquid state even at room temperature. Some examples of these are oils derived from nuts, salmon, avocado, peanut butter, and olive oil, just to mention a few.

Beneficial Proteins versus Detrimental Proteins

Do you belong to the group of individuals who associate the term protein with robust muscular development and a well-defined abdominal region? Indeed, protein plays a crucial role in facilitating the growth and development of muscular tissues. Additionally, it enhances physiological processes, augments physical prowess, and fosters daily vitality. This is the reason why it is imperative to maintain an adequate protein intake within your dietary regimen.

Consuming an appropriate quantity of protein will prove advantageous. Indulging excessively or consuming insufficient quantities is not advisable. Additionally, it is pertinent for you to be cognizant of the existence of two distinct protein types. There exists a category of proteins that confer beneficial effects on health, while there also exist sources of proteins that should be judiciously consumed or completely avoided.

The thing about protein is that to know whether or not it is good, you should take a look at its nutrient base. Additionally, it is essential to be cognizant of the sourcing process, which entails examining the methods employed in the animal's upbringing and farming practices. Additional factors to take into account encompass the inclusion of omega-3 fatty acids and the presence of saturated fat in the aforementioned.

It is essential to also consider that animal meat is not the sole source of protein accessible in the present day. Plant-derived soy is present. It contains a wealth of nutrients and possesses beneficial properties that promote gastrointestinal health. Additionally, a variety of grains, legumes, and even vegetables can provide ample amounts of protein. Portobello mushrooms, in particular, boast exceptional protein content.

Elucidating Misunderstandings Regarding Carbohydrates and Lipids

One of the lesser acknowledged truths in the field of nutrition is that fats possess a significantly higher caloric value than carbohydrates, with a ratio of 9 to 4.

Having acquired this knowledge, you may be interested in exploring the reason behind the prominence of carbohydrates as the primary source of glucose, despite the fact that fats possess a significantly higher caloric ratio.

The crux of the matter revolves around the examination of how the human body metabolizes calories derived from fat in contrast to the metabolic processes involved in processing calories obtained from carbohydrates.

The primary finding elucidates that the human body demonstrates enhanced and expedited extraction of ATP from carbohydrates, surpassing the efficiency exhibited in the extraction process from fats or any other dietary sources.

The more basic the carbohydrates, the quicker your body synthesizes ATP. A roster of simple carbohydrates would encompass refined flour products, unprocessed sugar, and fruit juice, whereas a compilation of complex carbohydrates would encompass leafy greens and whole grains.

Complex carbohydrates, analogous to fats, tend to undergo metabolism at a slower rate compared to simple carbohydrates.

Consequently, consumption of a serving of carbohydrates leads to an instantaneous elevation in the individual's blood glucose level.

The abrupt elevation in blood glucose levels will instigate a rapid discharge of substantial quantities of insulin. The insulin triggers your body to begin absorbing glucose from the blood stream, potentially converting the glucose into fat.

The subsequent event in this sequence involves inducing a depletion of blood sugar levels, leading to a concurrent reduction in serotonin levels, thereby heightening the likelihood of experiencing fatigue, lethargy, and an increased sensation of hunger.

The result of this carbohydrate-induced roller coaster journey is indulging in snacks.

The rapid increase and subsequent decline in carbohydrates and sugar levels lead to the commencement of snacking, ultimately causing you to surpass or exceed your AMR target.

One notable benefit of incorporating fats into your diet and not completely eliminating them is their ability to gradually release sugars into the bloodstream as compared to carbohydrates.

The advantage of fats exhibiting a reduced rate of release is the provision of a consistent and enduring source of energy, devoid of subsequent episodes of sudden depletion commonly associated with consuming sugars.

Another advantage of fats is that they remain in the stomach for an extended period of time, resulting in prolonged digestion and a prolonged feeling of satiety.

Consumption of an optimal ratio of fats and carbohydrates elicits a deceleration in the digestive process of carbohydrates, concurrently augmenting the assimilation of essential nutrients that are derived from both fats and carbohydrates.

This brings me to the third advantage of fats. Dietary fats play a crucial role in the absorption of nutrients and vitamins.

This is the situation where any type of fad diet has the potential to disrupt your entire system.

Any dietary regimen that decreases fat intake, unless balanced by a substantial increase in carbohydrates, will significantly diminish the calorie supply necessary to sustain bodily function.

Opting to eliminate fat from your dietary intake results in experiencing a rapid and intense increase in sugar levels, while simultaneously depriving your body of essential nutrients.

It is crucial to remain cognizant of the fundamental health advantages encompassed by the consumption of fats in promoting and preserving one's overall well-being. Fat is an essential component in any well-rounded dietary regimen.

Italian Style Meatballs

- 1 tablespoon Italian Seasoning

- 1 1/2 cups clean tomato sauce

- 1/4 cup fresh, grated parmesan cheese

- 1 1/2 pounds lean, ground turkey

- 1 tablespoon garlic powder

- 1 tablespoon fresh onion powder

In an ample mixing bowl, combine the turkey with the spices and knead the mixture together.

Shape the meat into twenty-two meatballs of walnut size and arrange them in a single layer within your slow cooker, which should ideally have a capacity of five quarts.

Carefully distribute the tomato sauce across the surface, ensuring that the meatballs are adequately and uniformly coated.

Distribute the cheese evenly over the surface, then adjust the setting of the slow cooker to low heat and allow it to cook for a duration of 4 hours.

Present the dish atop a bed of pasta, accompanied by a liberal sprinkling of parmesan cheese.

Recipes For Wholesome Pizza Muffins

- 1stick Cold Butter, cut into cubes

- 3/4 Cup Monterey Jack Cheese, cubed (mozzarella works as well)

- 2/3 Cup Applegate Farms pepperoni, cut into quarters

- 1 Egg

- 3/4 Cup Buttermilk

- 1/4 Cup Water

- 1 1/2 Cups Whole Wheat Flour

- 1 1/2 Cups Oat Flour

- 2Tbl Tapioca Starch(arrowroot will work as well)

- 1/2 tsp Sea Salt

- 1/4 tsp Fresh onion Powder

- 1   1/2   tsp   Dried   Italian Seasoning(oregano, parsley, basil)

- 1 1/2 Tsp Baking Powder

Set the oven temperature to 400° F and coat the muffin tins with grease.

Employ a mixing bowl and combine tapioca starch, whole wheat flour, herbs, oat flour, fresh onion powder, salt, and baking powder utilizing a whisk.

Incorporate diced butter into the mixture, using your fingertips, until it resembles coarse crumbs.

Incorporate pepperoni and cheese into the mixture, ensuring thorough distribution.

Obtain another bowl and proceed to incorporate buttermilk, egg, and water into it. Incorporate the mixture into the dry ingredients and thoroughly combine using a spatula until a cohesive dough is achieved.

Utilizing a generously sized scoop, carefully distribute the mixture evenly into the individual wells of the muffin tin, ensuring there are 12 equal portions.

Place in a preheated oven and bake for a duration of 10 to 12 minutes.

Take out from the oven and allow to cool for a duration of two minutes.

It is advisable to retain the item within a hermetically-sealed receptacle.

Mango Chicken

4 minced garlic cloves

¼ tsp. ginger

1 mango diced

¼ tsp. pepper

3 tomatoes

2 ½ c. water

1 c. brown rice

2 tsp. salsa

2 Tbsp. sesame seeds

1 lb. chicken breast

1 tsp. olive oil

Directions:

Retrieve a saucepan and proceed to bring the salsa and water to a boiling point. Incorporate the rice and allow it to simmer for a duration of 25 minutes to ensure thorough cooking.

The sesame seeds should be toasted in a skillet until they attain a golden hue. Distribute evenly onto a plate to allow for cooling.

Add a generous amount of oil to the pan, followed by the addition of the chicken. Add the pepper, ginger, and garlic for seasoning, and cook for a duration of 4 minutes until thoroughly cooked.

Place the mango into the pan and gently distribute it among the chicken using a spoon. Proceed to sauté the ingredients for a duration of 2 minutes, following which you can incorporate the lime juice and tomatoes into the mixture and allow it to simmer for a period of 5 minutes.

Please place this on top of the rice and savor the dish.

Japanese Style Meatball Soup

Ingredients

Meatballs

8 ounces fresh broccoli florets

8 ounces baby carrots, cut in half diagonally

2 (3 ounce) packages oriental-flavor instant ramen noodles

6 ounces fresh sugar snap peas, stems and strings removed

2 teaspoons dark oriental sesame oil

Sliced scallion (for garnish)

8 ounces lean ground beef

1/4 cup dry breadcrumbs

1 large egg white

1 tablespoon minced fresh ginger

1/2 tablespoon light soy sauce

2 teaspoons minced garlic

Soup

Directions

To prepare meatballs, combine the ingredients and evenly spread the mixture onto a sheet of wax paper. Gently shape the mixture into a square and proceed to cut it into thirty-six equally sized squares.

Please bring a large pot to a boil, using five cups of water.

Add in carrots.

Cook, with a lid in place, for a duration of 5 minutes or until the desired state of tenderness is achieved.

Place the meatballs into the cooking vessel. Incorporate the contents of the noodle seasoning packets.

Mix in broccoli.

Reduce the temperature to a gentle simmer and cover the dish, allowing the vegetables to soften for a duration of 7 minutes.

Subsequently, divide each block of noodles into four equal parts and incorporate them into the soup.

Prepare the dish, by stirring to disentangle the strands, for a duration of 60 seconds.

Incorporate sugar snap peas into the mixture and simmer for a duration of 120 seconds (equivalent to 2 minutes) or until the noodles attain a tender consistency and the peas achieve a vibrant green hue.

Incorporate sesame oil and remove from the source of heat.

Incorporate the scallions as a decorative topping within the bowls.

The Expenditures Associated With Maintaining A Healthy Diet

Adopting the clean eating lifestyle entails numerous advantages, primarily pertaining to one's health. Nevertheless, in order to partake in these benefits, there are various expenses which individuals must bear. Attaining holistic well-being necessitates striking a balance between short-term gains and long-term benefits.

This lifestyle incurs only a single financial expense. As the adoption of a clean eating lifestyle entails emphasizing the consumption of unprocessed, organic foods, individuals can anticipate a certain elevation in their expenditures on groceries. It is widely acknowledged that high-quality cuisine often comes with a considerable price tag, yet the value provided by these ingredients justifies the expenditure. Whilst the adoption of this lifestyle entails higher expenses associated with the quality of food, there exist various approaches through which these expenses may be offset.

As individuals embark upon the act of meal preparation in their households and subsequently consume said meals within the confines of their homes, they curtail superfluous expenditures on food items procured from external sources such as takeout establishments and the like. In addition to cost savings, they are accumulating substantial amount of savings. Typically, the prices of food items in restaurants see a significant mark-up of around 400 percent on average. The identical type of cuisine, crafted using premium ingredients within the confines of one's own residence, is available at a significantly reduced price compared to its market value.

An alternative approach to managing food expenditures would involve sourcing from nearby suppliers and favoring ingredients that are in season. Local farmers' markets provide high-quality produce at more affordable prices compared to supermarket chains. One noteworthy aspect is that these products are sourced directly from agricultural establishments, enabling consumers to procure them directly from the cultivators.

Adopting this specific lifestyle will necessitate a certain expenditure of time as well. Altering long-standing habits can prove to be a considerable challenge. It will require a considerable period for individuals to acclimate themselves to the dietary options available to them, gaining proficiency in meal preparation within their own homes, strategically organizing meals and adhering to them, incorporating physical activity into their routines, and even diverting from the consumption of unhealthy foods which they may have indulged in on a daily basis. This entails a minor concession to reap the enduring advantages associated with adhering to a healthy diet.

Upon investing their monetary resources and time into the endeavor, individuals promptly receive compensation in the shape of healthcare savings. Health savings refer to the accumulated funds resulting from reduced expenses on medical treatments or prescription drugs. As an individual enhances their dietary practices, their general well-being undergoes improvement, leading to a stronger and more balanced physique, with a reduced susceptibility of the immune system to harmful stimuli.

Consequently, this leads to a decrease in the incidence of illnesses, consequently resulting in a substantial diminishment in the requirement for medical intervention. Medical expenses, particularly in cases where individuals lack sufficient insurance coverage, have the potential to incur annual costs in the thousands of dollars. When individuals are able to reduce their expenditures on healthcare, they simultaneously enhance their prospects for increased income through employment. Reduced instances of absenteeism result in increased presence in the workplace, ultimately contributing to larger remuneration on a monthly basis.

The Daily Ingestion Of Detrimental Toxins

In the present time, it has become challenging to prepare a meal for oneself without encountering various cautionary notifications regarding potential food hazards." One can substantially mitigate the chances of serving harmful ingredients by thoroughly examining the labels, acquiring knowledge about the origin of food, and maintaining a kitchen environment devoid of such undesirable food constituents as much as feasible. It is crucial to emphasize the significance of this practice when deliberating on the dietary choices made for your children. This is primarily attributable to the fact that, due to their smaller stature, they consume ingredients in a proportionately higher amount compared to adults.

The subsequent list comprises various toxins that individuals should refrain from encountering:

Pesticides

These substances are utilized in the process of treating fruits and vegetables, acting as toxins that eliminate unwanted garden pests prior to any potential damage they may cause to the crop or harvest. Regrettably, these pesticides often result in the presence of residues. Despite the mandatory screening and safety assessments that all produce must undergo prior to being sold, numerous individuals opt to steer clear entirely of even the most minute traces of residues.

Health Hazards: carcinogenic effects; dermatological irritation; disruption of endocrine system; impairment of nervous system.

Affected Food Items: Fruits and vegetables cultivated from the soil, specifically apples, peaches, nectarines, strawberries, grapes, celery, spinach, sweet bell peppers, cucumbers, cherry tomatoes, snap peas, potatoes, hot peppers, and kale.

Proposed solution: It is imperative that organic food products conform to strict standards regarding the absence of synthetic pesticides. Therefore, it is highly recommended to seek out organic alternatives.

Butylated Hydroxyanisole (BHA) and Butylated Hydroxytoluene (BHT)

These additives are frequently used as preservatives in commercially manufactured food products that are readily available in supermarkets, sandwich bars, and various other retail establishments that offer convenient pre-packaged meals or grab-and-go food options.

Health Hazards: Onset of Cancer; disruption of endocrine system; adverse effects on male reproductive health; compromised blood coagulation capabilities

Affected Food Items: chewing gum; butter; cereals; snack foods; beer; cereals; other food products containing fats and oils

Resolution: Examine the ingredient lists on food packaging labels as a measure to circumvent these deleterious toxins.

Recombinant Bovine Somatotropin (rBST)

This synthetically-created endocrine substance is administered to bovines with the objective of augmenting their lactation capacity. It has been demonstrated that there is a notable augmentation of insulin-like growth factor-1 (IGF-1) in dairy products.

Health Hazards: cancers affecting the breast, prostate, and colon.

Impacted Food Items: Dairy products, including milk, cheese, and butter.

Resolution: Opt for dairy products that are organic or free from rBGH.

Sodium Aluminium Sulphate and Potassium Aluminium Sulphate

Numerous packaged commodities, such as cheese items, bakery products, and microwave popcorn, consist of these substances. They serve as additives employed for the purpose of modulating the acidity levels of food products, albeit they have been recognized as toxins due to their capacity to potentially induce other deleterious health conditions.

Health Hazards: Adverse impacts on reproductive, neurological, behavioral, and developmental functions.

Foods Impacted: Potable water; sodium bicarbonate; analgesics such as paracetamol and aspirin; certain types of fruits and vegetables; wheat flour; dairy products; confections.

Solution: Take the necessary precautionary measure of thoroughly examining ingredient lists in order to prevent exposure to this harmful substance.

Bisphenol-A (BPA)

This chemical is frequently encountered in the inner linings of beverage cans and bottles, primarily attributed to its affordability and convenient production process. Additionally, its characteristics bear resemblance to certain hormones present in the human body.

Health Hazards: breast or prostate carcinoma; reproductive disorders; behavioral abnormalities; overweight; diabetes

Affected Food Items: Canned food products and beverages; bottled beverages; plastic food storage containers

Solution: Avoid canned foods. Please opt for fresh, dried, or frozen alternatives instead. Choose glass, porcelain, or stainless steel alternatives in lieu of plastic containers.

Sodium Nitrite/Nitrate

Food additives employed as preservatives to inhibit the proliferation of pathogenic bacteria, commonly utilized in deli products such as processed meats.

Health Hazards: Diverse forms of cancer.

Affected food items include various meats such as bacon, ham, sausages, and hot dogs.

Resolution: To circumvent the presence of this toxic substance, it is advisable to carefully peruse the ingredient lists. Exercise caution when consuming products labeled as 'uncured' or 'no added nitrites/nitrates'. Frequently, they opt for celery juice as a substitute, given its elevated nitrate content.

Polycyclic Aromatic Hydrocarbons

When the process of combustion or exposure to highly elevated temperatures occurs, these substances are produced as a result of fat being consumed.

Health Hazards: Formation of tumors; development of cancer; impaired reproductive health; heightened risk of obesity; manifestation of skin and blood disorders; compromised immune system;

Foods Impacted: Any water, sustenance, particulate matter, or emissions that become in contact with heated fatty substances; can also arise from hydrocarbons, waste combustion, domestic heating units, and vehicle motors.

Alternative: "Remedy: Prior to grilling, it is advisable to partially cook the meats, followed by placing them on the barbecue at a lower heat setting. This approach ensures that the extremely high temperatures necessary for toxin formation are effectively averted."

Heterocyclic Amines

Another chemical residue, resulting from the chemical reactions that occur between specific compounds present in various types of muscle meats when exposed to high temperatures, such as those occurring during grilling.

Health Risks: Cancer

Food Products Impacted: Beef, pork, ham, fish, poultry, lamb — any kind of meat that consists of muscular tissue and is subjected to high temperatures through grilling, barbecuing, broiling, or other similar methods of cooking.

Resolution: Prior to grilling, barbecuing, or broiling, it is advisable to partially cook the meats and subsequently complete the process over a gentle heat, thereby preventing the occurrence of elevated temperatures that may induce the formation of this harmful substance.

Acrylamide

This compound is generated through the process of cooking or frying starchy foods such as grains and potatoes at elevated temperatures.

Health Hazards: Carcinogenic effects; neuropathy; dermal irritations.

Affected Food Items: White rice, potatoes, corn, wheat, pasta

Resolution: It is advisable to refrain from consuming deep-fried food items, such as potato chips, crackers, toasted cereals, cookies, and bread crusts.

Bromination of Vegetable Oil

This additive, which is incorporated into select fruit-flavored soft drinks and sodas, serves the purpose of inhibiting the occurrence of ingredient separation upon settling of the liquid.

Health Hazards: Reproductive ailments; behavioral impairments

Impacted Food Items: Fruit-infused beverages

Resolution: Examine the ingredients listed on the label.

Synthetic Food Colorants

These substances are employed to bestow a distinct hue upon numerous food and beverage items, typically with the intent of establishing an association with a different entity (such as the color of strawberries in strawberry-flavored ice cream).

Potential Health Hazards: Neurological impairments like attention deficit hyperactivity disorder (ADHD), increased hyperactivity, and migraines; heightened anxiety; and increased susceptibility to cancer.

Impacted Food Products: Numerous confectioneries; beverages; frozen treats; desserts; dairy products; condiments; chewing products.

Resolution: Engage in the diligent practice of perusing ingredient labels to circumvent potential concerns.

Regarding the matter of Dioxins

These substances are classified as toxic pollutants, originating from various natural and artificial combustion processes, subsequently being assimilated into the organisms' biological systems. They exhibit solubility in lipids and organic solvents, thus can be found within lipid-rich food products.

Potential Health Hazards: Adverse effects on reproduction and development; compromised immune function; disrupted hormone levels; increased susceptibility to cancer.

Affected Foods: Any food made from animals that contains a portion of naturally occurring fats.

Resolution: Opt for food options that contain minimal amounts of fat or are completely devoid of fat.

Organisms that have been genetically modified (GM organisms)

Genetically modified organisms (GMOs) are living entities, including plants and animals, that have undergone genetic alterations with the aim of enhancing specific traits such as resistance to diseases or tolerance to pesticides.

Potential Health Hazards: Impaired organ function; digestive system disturbances; compromised immune system; expedited aging process; reduced fertility

Affected Food Groups: Numerous processed food items that utilize ingredients derived from corn, soy, cottonseed, canola, and sugar beet.

Proposed solution: Embrace organic products! Certified organic foods offer a guaranteed assurance of being free from genetically modified organisms (GMOs). As GMO labeling is not mandatory, choosing organic is crucial for effectively sidestepping the presence of GMOs.

Principles For Achieving Optimal Health And Maintaining Physical Fitness

Considering the multitude of hazards linked to the accumulation of excessive fat in the body, maintaining a healthy and proportionate body weight in relation to your height can greatly contribute to your overall well-being. Exercise caution in preserving a healthy BMI within acceptable parameters. Maintain optimal muscle to fat ratios and ensure a healthy body composition to promote longevity and personal fulfillment.

Objective establishment: Prior to initiating the development of a fitness training program, it is imperative to establish specific goals, as this will enhance your dedication and adherence to the regimen. By employing the practice of goal setting, one gains the ability to clearly discern their desired outcomes, comprehend the underlying motivations, and crucially determine the precise strategies required to accomplish said objectives. When setting objectives, it is imperative to formulate both immediate and ultimate goals. Your objectives will serve as your compass as you embark on a transformative path towards weight reduction and physical well-being.

Engage in sincere self-reflection: Take into account your schedule and present life situation. If you have plans to embark on a significant project at your workplace or have upcoming extensive travel planned in the coming months, it may be prudent to delay until you can truly devote your attention to the program. Failure may result from a lack of commitment and dedication to exert maximum effort during exercise sessions.

Exercise: One must prioritize and bear in mind the significance of incorporating physical activity into one's lifestyle, as it plays a crucial role in weight management, overall fitness, and the preservation of one's overall well-being and health. Every physician consistently places great emphasis on the significance of engaging in regular physical activity. The extent of physical activity is inconsequential as long as you take the initial initiative. One can initiate their fitness regimen by engaging in leisurely strolls or jogs, allocating approximately 30 minutes per day. Eventually, as the body adapts to such physical activity, one can gradually incorporate more vigorous exercises. Adopting a regimen of physical activity and adhering to a nutritious diet should be the lifestyle modifications you prioritize, as they are sure to yield long-term benefits that you will not repent.

Addressing your stress levels: The presence of anxiety and stress can contribute to various health complications, spanning from cardiovascular disorders to gastrointestinal ailments. A considerable number of individuals are uninformed of the appropriate means to manage their anxiety. Contemplation, physical activity, engaging in passions, cultivating a sense of spirituality, connecting with the natural environment, establishing suitable limits, and pursuing enjoyable pastimes can all aid in mitigating the adverse physiological consequences of stress. Make an effort to avoid overexertion during work. Incorporate intermittent intervals of rest, brief retreats, designated periods of leave, and similar measures while ensuring you are surrounded by individuals who provide you with unwavering support.

Staying Hydrated: Throughout the course of the day, your body will expend a significant amount of its water supply to regulate its internal temperature through perspiration. Therefore, it is crucial to regularly replenish your body with water to maintain optimal hydration. Do not consume carbonated beverages or juices that contain refined sugars or high fructose corn syrup ('HFCS'), as these ingredients contribute empty calories that can result in the accumulation of stubborn, hard-to-eliminate body fat. Employ fresh, unadulterated fruits with water to infuse flavor into your water.

If you opt to consume a glass of water as the initial morning routine, you will effectively stimulate your digestive system, promoting the combustion of persistent adipose tissue. It is advisable to consume 4-6 servings of water per day.

Rejuvenation: The state of rest has a profound impact on both our physical and emotional welfare. A substantial number of individuals suffer from inadequate rest, which consequently contributes to the adoption of unhealthy lifestyles. The lack of sufficient rest significantly impacts the digestive system, cognitive function, focus, cardiovascular health, and the regulation of stress hormones. Repose enables the body to undergo recuperation, repair, and restoration in a manner that is fundamentally unachievable during wakefulness. By means of relaxation, there is an augmentation in metabolism, a crucial factor in facilitating the maintenance of a well-balanced body weight.

Swimming

Continual exercise on the treadmill or elliptical can be quite demanding when the weather resembles the torrid conditions of the sixth circle of Dante's Inferno. Swimming is widely regarded as an exceptionally effective means by which individuals can maintain their physical fitness. This is primarily attributed to the fact that it provides an enjoyable means of participating in physical exercise. One of the advantageous aspects of swimming is its inherent capacity to produce a comprehensive impact on the human physique. As a result, allocating a portion of your time to engage in swimming activities not only facilitates weight reduction, but also contributes to overall revitalization. If you are seeking an engaging approach to achieving weight loss, consider incorporating swimming into your routine.

Modes Of Commencing A Clean Eating Regimen

If you possess a strong desire to adopt a clean eating routine, it is imperative that you assess and amend your dietary practices. By taking these initial measures to attentively monitor your food choices, you will gradually witness a seamless transition and eventually find it ingrained as a natural habit, necessitating minimal exertion. What course of action should be taken initially?

Embark on your journey towards embracing a clean eating lifestyle by visiting the local market. The preceding chapter shall serve as your current reference. Ensure you have it readily available while making purchases, marking the completion of the initial stage.

Commence preparing your meals independently. Why subject yourself to the torment of uncertainty surrounding the ingredients incorporated into the aforementioned spaghetti sauce, when you have the option to prepare it in the comfort of your own abode, utilizing fresh tomatoes, herbs, and spices? Time is no excuse here, as in most of the cases, you will have to spend this allegedly "saved" time at the doctor's office. Hence, in order to mitigate the adverse outcome, it is more advisable to allocate time to the culinary domain as opposed to being confined within the confines of a medical facility.

Reduce alcohol consumption. Purifying your body requires ensuring the cleanliness of your beverage intake. This should not be interpreted as a suggestion to entirely refrain from alcohol; however, it is imperative to substantially minimize its consumption as an essential component of a meticulous routine. Please adhere to the same regulations pertaining to beverage consumption and refrain from ingesting excessive calories through drinks; instead, consider obtaining these calories from solid food sources, particularly carbohydrates. According to scientific research, it has been demonstrated that carbohydrates consumed in conjunction with beverages are metabolized at a faster rate and undergo more intense combustion compared to those ingested alongside solid food.

UN-sweeten your diet. Lactose, dextrose, sucrose, glucose, and starch are various types of sugar that manufacturers of sweet products refine, manipulate, and modify meticulously in order to stimulate your reward system and foster addiction. However, if you are unable to control your desire for sweet foods, it would be prudent to appease it by consuming fresh grapes, natural honey, or unsweetened dates.

Opt for whole grains instead of refined grains, as they encompass the germ, endosperm, and bran components. They serve as excellent sources of dietary fiber, essential minerals, and a variety of crucial nutrients, including but not limited to potassium, magnesium, and calcium. Therefore, enhance your dietary intake by incorporating brown rice, barley, quinoa, and oats, which will result in significantly improved well-being.

Enhance your diet by incorporating a variety of fresh fruits and vegetables. Vegetables serve as an excellent reservoir of essential vitamins, while also maintaining a low caloric content, rendering them amenable to generous portions without causing concern for one's body weight. It is unnecessary to emphasize their significant relevance for the skin, blood vessels, heart, bones, and muscle tissue.

Choose meat wisely. When making a purchase of meat from a retail establishment, it is advisable to inquire with the butcher regarding the diet of the animal, specifically whether it was fed a grass-centric or grain-centric diet. Every reputable supermarket management possesses the requisite certifications that provide explicit documentation of the animals' feed and enable transparency in providing consumers with this information. It is recommended to refrain from consuming grain-fed beef or frozen beef patties. In terms of the veal and pork, they ought to exhibit a modest level of moisture, a subtle grayish pink hue, and possess a resilient texture. The presence of vivid red or deep purple pigment serves as a testament to the chemical processing that the meat has been subjected to. Pork chops, roasted lamb, hamburgers, and minced beef are not optimal selections. Ultimately, it is advisable to substitute all smoked, cured, or salted meat options, such as ham, bacon, salami, pastrami, hot dogs, or sausages, with fresh meat alternatives. By doing so, one can explore the realm of making appetizing and nourishing meat-based dishes at home through the utilization of natural spices, herbs, and vegetables.

Ensure that your body receives the requisite quantity of water. You may be weary of hearing this, notwithstanding the pivotal significance of water in cleansing your body. It is highly advisable to refrain from exerting oneself to consume excessive amounts of water if one does not feel the need for it. However, intermittently sipping water ensures that one's body remains in a conditioned, hydrated, and invigorated state. You have the option to enhance the flavor of your water by incorporating fresh fruits or berries, but it is advisable to refrain from including any sweeteners in order to minimize caloric intake. For instance, fresh lemon-infused water can effectively rejuvenate and invigorate you throughout the course of the day.

By critically examining your dietary patterns and substituting previous choices with more nutritious and hygienic alternatives, you will witness and derive gratification from the outcomes within an exceptionally brief timeframe. Our bodies are inherently receptive and thankful, thus prioritize nourishing oneself with wholesome foods to attain physical and mental well-being.

www.ingramcontent.com/pod-product-compliance
Lightning Source LLC
Chambersburg PA
CBHW071212020426
42333CB00015B/1384